NO MORE TICS!

Help for Tic Disorders,
Tourette Syndrome, TikTok Tics and More

GW00503632

SARAH CHANA RADCLIFFE, M.Ed., C. Psych

No More Tics!

Help for Tic Disorders, Tourette Syndrome, TikTok Tics and More!

© by 2021 Sarah Chana Radcliffe

All rights reserved. The use of any part of this publication reproduced, transmitted in any form or by any means, electronic, mechanical, photocopying, recording, or otherwise, or stored in a retrieval system, without the prior written consent of the publisher is an infringement of the copyright law.

Interior and Cover design by Daniel J. Eyenegho

ISBN: 9798786108690

CONTENTS

To my husband Avraham,

without whose encouragement and support

this book would not have been written.

Many thanks go to Deena Weinberg

for her careful reading of the manuscript,

her extremely helpful suggestions and her thoughtful editing.

DISCLAIMER

The information in this book is for informational purposes only and is not intended to replace the advice or recommendations of a psychological or medical practitioner. Do not use this book to diagnose or treat health conditions; consult your doctor or other qualified health professional regarding diagnosis and treatment of your own or your child's health condition and the advisability of undertaking a self-help program. The author disclaims any liability in connection with the use of this information and makes no representations or warranties with respect to the accuracy, completeness, or fitness for a particular purpose of this book and excludes all liability to the extent permitted by law for any errors or omissions and for any loss, damage, harm or expense (whether direct or indirect) suffered by anyone relying on any information contained in this book.

CHAPTER ONE
TICS - WHAT THEY ARE AND WHAT THEY AREN'T

Do you - or perhaps your child, partner or someone else you care about - make unwanted sounds or movements? Have you received a diagnosis of "Tic Disorder" or "Tourette's Disorder"? Or maybe there hasn't been an official diagnosis at this point, but you're aware that something is going on (twitches, blinking, touching, coughing, throat clearing, squeaking, bending, twisting or something else) that really shouldn't be. You've been assuming that you can, if you try hard enough, make it go away. If the problem belongs to your child or partner, you might have found yourself routinely telling that person to "stop doing that" in hopes of retraining what appears to be an annoying habit.

In fact, you might have assumed that the behavior in question was what we call a "nervous habit" even if your doctor already called it a tic. But the truth is that nervous habits are different from tics. Nervous habits - like drumming our fingers on the table or swinging our legs while sitting in a chair, rubbing our forehead or biting our nails, are all repetitive behaviors that help regulate the nervous system by either calming us down when we're agitated or stimulating us when we're bored. Like tics, these seemingly unnecessary sounds and movements often annoy those around us.

And like tics, nervous habits, bad habits and all kinds of other habits, aren't usually successfully eradicated through reprimands. But if you were able to stop your own "nervous habit" by sheer willpower or if you were able to get your child or spouse to stop theirs through reminders, complaints or threats, then this is a sign that what you were dealing with was possibly a nervous habit but definitely *not* a tic. Cracking one's knuckles, picking one's nose, and twirling one's hair are all examples of nervous habits that can be stopped through *conscious intention* when motivation is high enough. Tics aren't like that. But interestingly, there are many other kinds of habits besides nervous habits. These, too, can be distinguished from tics based on their receptivity to conscious intervention. We'll look at some of these below.

For now, let's just note that tics are **involuntary** behaviors - something like hiccups. Just as we don't intentionally hiccup, we don't intentionally perform a tic. Moreover, just as we can't tell ourselves NOT to hiccup, we can't tell ourselves not to tic (although we can sometimes delay it a bit). Tics are something that happen *to* us, within us - that's why they're called "involuntary."

Moreover, tic movements and sounds serve no apparent purpose. They don't relieve anxiety or calm our nervous system. They don't bring relief from stress. They are neurological phenomena caused by a disturbance in the movement center of the brain, caused either by genetic conditions at birth (tic disorders that run in families most commonly appear in children between the ages of 5 and 10, with the most common ages of onset being 7 or 8) or by external conditions. For instance, tics can sometimes be triggered from brain reactions to drugs (such as antipsychotic medications, cocaine and amphetamines) or from illness (such as strep infections) or from diseases (such as cerebral palsy or Huntington's Disease). To be even more precise, it has been posited that tics are the result of dysfunction in the basal ganglia and cortico-striato-thalamo circuits in the brain as well as a dysfunction in the dopaminergic system co-existing with GABAergic inhibition. That's a fancy medical way to say that tics are caused by something very physical going on in the brain! Some scientists believe that the brain issues that lead to tics can also be triggered by external factors such as prenatal conditions, food sensitivities, environmental toxins, emotional stress and other aspects of our modern world.

The bottom line is that we don't DO tics; tics *happen* to us and they do so because of brain processes. It may now seem that everything is clear and that you can diagnose yourself or your loved one as having, or not having, a tic disorder, based on whether it can be cured with willpower. But alas, you don't yet have enough information to make your diagnosis. In fact, tics are so confusing that many pediatricians, doctors and mental health professionals will fail to provide a correct initial diagnosis. Let's see why.

Tics and Tic-Look-Alikes

We've already acknowledged that there is something called a nervous habit - a sound or movement we perform to help balance and calm our nervous system. We should also note that a specific tic can certainly look the same as a regular nervous habit. But to make matters even more confusing, a specific tic can look exactly the same as a compulsive behavior that is found in a condition called obsessive-compulsive disorder (OCD). For example, small repetitive movements like tapping or turning can be seen in both Tic Disorder and in OCD. Counting, touching things a certain way or a certain number of times, saying things, washing, checking, moving in certain ways, and thinking in certain patterns are additional common examples of obsessive behaviors (also called compulsions or rituals), some of which resemble complex tics to the outside observer.

Unlike tic behaviors, OCD behaviors *aren't* involuntary - they are performed intentionally - sort of. In OCD, a person feels *compelled* to perform certain behaviors (to the sufferers, it doesn't *feel* like they have a choice), but when motivation is high, people with OCD CAN actually refrain from doing the repetitive action. This ability to exert conscious control forms the basis of the evidenced-based treatment for OCD which is called CBT - cognitive-behavioral therapy. By changing thoughts and behaviors, and in many cases by also addressing underlying traumatic stress, a person with OCD can stop performing repetitive sounds or movements. Normally, OCD sufferers don't discover the voluntary nature of their actions until they begin treatment. Once they receive the proper help, they find that they can profoundly decrease their performance of repetitive actions, and in milder cases, remove them altogether.

However, the voluntary aspect of OCD behaviors is not all that we need to understand. We need to understand the *motivational* differences between OCD behaviors and the tic behaviors we find in Tic Disorders. You see, even though people with OCD CAN stop performing their behaviors, they may not WANT to stop performing them because those behaviors serve a purpose. Typically, OCD rituals stave off a painful emotion such as dread or fear of death or terror of something awful happening. Performing the behavior can distract a person from those painful emotions and in some cases, may even be experienced in a superstitious way, as a preventative measure designed to ensure that nothing bad will occur.

Because the behaviors relieve the person of intense negative feelings - even if only momentarily - they are addictive. The OCD sufferer turns to them again and again (and typically, more and more often) to ease anxiety.

Tics, however, do NOT bring momentary relief from painful emotions. They serve no psychological purpose whatsoever. Tic sufferers are usually more than happy to give them up because they receive no benefit from these sounds or movements.

More Tic-Look-Alikes

We humans love our habits and so there are plenty more. Trichotillomania, Excoriation Disorder (Dermatillomania), Onychophagia (nail biting), and Onychotillomania (obsessive nail picking or finger sucking) are three other disorders that look like Tic Disorders. Or, some would say that they look like OCD. They certainly look like bad habits! Trichotillomania is the habit of mindlessly pulling out one's hair, eyebrows or eyelashes. Excoriation Disorder involves mindlessly picking at one's skin or scabs on one's skin, and the nail habit disorders involve compulsively picking at, rubbing or sucking the area in and around the nails or biting one's nails. And there are even more BFRB (body-focused repetitive behaviors) listed in the DSM-5 (Mental Health Diagnostic Manual) such as lip-biting disorder, tongue chewing disorder and trichophagia (compulsive hair eating disorder). All of these habits respond to treatment in similar ways to the habits of OCD. Once brought to consciousness and addressed in professional treatment - which can include medication, lifestyle adjustments, psychotherapy and behavior therapy - they can be significantly reduced and in some cases, eliminated. These habits come under conscious control. Again, not so with tics.

Because we might be engaging in a repetitive movement for a variety of reasons, outside observers such as parents and other family members, are going to have a lot of trouble understanding what it is we're doing and why. To highlight how difficult it is to identify a Tic Disorder just by observing it, let's consider the following example:

Imagine that there are five people sitting in the waiting room of a medical clinic: Josh, Mitch, Abe, Aaron and Max. As he reads his magazine, Josh is moving his finger rhythmically and repetitively back and forth along the arm of the chair he's sitting in. He has an internal drive to make that particular movement because he has a Tic Disorder. Mitch, a person with OCD, is making the same movement on the arm of his chair but he's also silently counting how many times he makes the movement; he needs to move his hand exactly 9 consecutive times in repetitive sets in order to calm his anxiety that something bad is about to happen. The third fellow, Abe, is making the identical movement on his chair but he's doing it because his ADHD makes him feel antsy while waiting and he just needs to move his body to discharge excess energy. Aaron is mindlessly rubbing his finger along the arm of his chair as he worries about his upcoming meeting with the doctor - his movement is one of his GAD-induced (Generalized Anxiety Disorder) "nervous habits" meant to calm his worried mind and help shake down his stress. Finally, there's Max sitting in the fifth chair, rubbing his finger along the upholstery. Max doesn't have a Tic Disorder, OCD, ADHD or Anxiety - he's a touchy-feely guy who just likes to rub his finger along the chair!

No one watching these five fellows would be able to identify the underlying cause of their finger movements. Their behavior would have to be thoroughly assessed in order to arrive at a correct diagnosis. This is why you probably want a good diagnostician to help you figure out what is actually going on in your own case of unwanted sounds and/or movements. Keep in mind that a correct diagnosis leads to the right treatment and an incorrect diagnosis leads to the wrong treatment. When the right person conducts a psychological interview, the right questions are asked. For instance, you may have no idea that your child is silently counting numbers or saying words as she makes repetitive movements. You probably wouldn't have known to inquire. The question comes out of professional psychological expertise, something that most parents lack. Unfortunately, incorrect assumptions can lead to delays in effective treatment for all of these disorders.

By the way, when it comes to Tic Disorders, a "good diagnostician" is most likely to be a neurologist, neuropsychologist or a neuropsychiatrist, rather than your general practitioner, pediatrician, psychotherapist, social worker, nurse or counseling psychologist. This is because Tic Disorders - as we've seen above - are neurological conditions that often accompany other psychiatric conditions such as OCD, ADHD, ASD (Autism Spectrum Disorder), Anxiety, LD (Learning Disabilities) and other neurological and psychiatric conditions. As we've noted, tics can also be triggered by illnesses, brain injury and medications. Brain doctors (neurologists) who are intimately familiar with all of these diagnoses are in the best position to recognize and accurately identify true tics and their underlying etiology through appropriate and extensive assessment. They can differentiate them from the behaviors that the same patient may be performing due to OCD, ADHD, BFRB and so on. Keep in mind that a person who has a Tic Disorder almost always has one or more of the "cousin" disorders (OCD, ADHD, Anxiety, LD etc.) as well. The diagnostician needs to be able to diagnose all of these conditions and separate them from each other. Effective treatment for Tic Disorders includes specific treatment for the tics *as well as* for the accompanying physical and mental health conditions.

Tics that come on *suddenly and intensely* are thought to be in a category of their own, a category requiring even more specialized diagnosis. These are the kind of tics that arise out of PANDAS or PANS (see detailed description of these conditions below) and are best assessed by specialists such as immunologists or those who are experts in the area of strep infections. These professionals will take blood tests and other diagnostic tests to determine the presence of streptococcal infections and other possible infections that can occur in the throat and many other areas of the body and that can trigger psychiatric and neurological disorders.

Tics and Tic Disorders

Let's take a closer look now at what constitutes a tic. Tics come in two main flavors: vocal tics and motor tics. Examples of vocal tics include:

- Grunts, sniffs, coughs, throat clearing, snorting, squeaks
- Repetition of words or phrases, or very rarely, an urge to repeat vulgar words (coprolalia)

Examples of motor tics include:

- Head jerking, head banging, shoulder shrugging
- Body twitching or jerking
- Nose wrinkling, sniffing, eye blinking, lip movements, grimacing, tongue movements
- Touching, grabbing or rubbing people or objects
- Hopping, jumping, bending, twisting

Tics range dramatically in their severity. They can be, and often are, so mild that they are hardly noticeable to outside observers. At the other extreme, tics can be so disruptive that they can cause intense emotional anguish, social dysfunction, and educational or occupational disability. Tics can be simple or complex, with simple tics being more common. Simple tics consist of one muscle group. An example would be coughing. Another example would be blinking. Complex tics involve several different muscle groups moving in a coordinated fashion. An example of a complex tic would be touching people. Another example would be repeating one's own words. A person's tics can change from simple to complex and from one muscle group to another ("He stopped touching people but now he is making squeaking noises.").

When people have both vocal and motor tics they will be diagnosed as having "Tourette Syndrome" (also called "Tourette's or TS"). If they only have one kind of tic (either motor or vocal) and the tic has persisted for more than a year, they will be diagnosed as having "Persistent Tic Disorder" (also called "Chronic Tic Disorder"). If the tics have been around for less than a year, they will usually receive the diagnosis of "Provisional Tic Disorder" (previously known as "Transient Tic Disorder").

As mentioned above, tics that have a very sudden and intense onset following a streptococcal (strep) infection may be diagnosed as PANDAS (Pediatric Autoimmune Neuropsychiatric Disorders Associated with Streptococcal Infections). A child whose tics are attributed to PANDAS may have either motor or vocal tics or both and usually also has an equally sudden and intense onset of symptoms of OCD, ADHD, Anxiety, Depression or other physical and/or mental health conditions.

Tics can also be caused by PANS (Pediatric Acute-Onset Neuropsychiatric Syndrome), which is a collection of auto-immune disorders that affect the brain but that are NOT associated with a strep infection.

TikTok Tics

In 2021, we witnessed the appearance of a new tic condition - a phenomenon referred to as TikTok Tics in the popular media and known in the medical community as Functional Neurological Disorder. These are tic movements (motor or vocal or both, and simple or complex) thought to be produced by cultural contagion - a psychological phenomenon that induces some form of physical or psychological illness in the masses (for a discussion of this process see the book "The Sleeping Beauties" by neurologist Dr. Suzanne O'Sullivan).

Teenagers - predominantly female - suddenly develop tic-type movements or sounds. At this point in time, there is a question about the etiology of these tics and whether they are actual tics created by the neurological conditions previously described or whether these are controllable behaviors and therefore indicative of some other condition. The question arises because these tics differ in many ways from the typical neurological tics we have described above, despite appearing identical. To begin with, they emerge most commonly in adolescence rather than at the age at which "normal" tics first appear (i.e. 6 - 8 yrs old). They happen more frequently in females whereas males are the gender most typically affected by regular tics. There is no "premonitory sensations" (urge) preceding these tics whereas there is an urge that precedes regular tics. Those who have these tics do not typically have the "cousin" conditions (ADHD, LD, OCD, etc) whereas other tic sufferers almost always do. Nor do these sufferers have a family history of tics, something which is highly characteristic of other tic sufferers. However what they DO have is a history of watching Tic behavior on social media (hence the name TikTok Tics).

As of the time of this writing, it is unclear whether those who are afflicted by the TikToc tics will be experiencing a temporary condition that will disappear on its own within a year (as occurs in Provisional Tic Disorder) or whether they will be experiencing a chronic condition (as happens in Persistent Tic Disorder). What is being considered by the professionals who are investigating TikTok Tics is that the condition might be the result of the stress perpetrated by the recent pandemic. For example, it might be a manifestation of, and reaction to, the psychological pressures endured by teens with sensitive brains who experienced intense social isolation at a critical point in their development. On the bright side, it appears that TikTok Tics do respond to the behavioral treatments available for regular tic disorders (see below) and therefore, it is quite likely that they will also respond well to the unique treatment protocol offered in this book, as will soon be explained.

CHAPTER TWO
TREATMENTS FOR TICS

Not all tics require treatment. Often tics aren't noticeable to anyone except closest family members and some aren't even noticed by them! Some tic sufferers themselves may not even realize that they have repetitive movements or that their personal behaviors or sounds are anything more than just quirky habits. In these cases, treatment may be unnecessary. These very mild Tic Disorders are not posing any real problems. In other cases, however, tics are annoying or disruptive enough that sufferers (or their families) definitely want an effective treatment to tame or cure them. Let's look at the available options for this second group.

The "Wait" Approach

Some pediatricians and other medical practitioners have a "wait it out" treatment approach for mild and moderate tics. When the tic sufferer is a child, this treatment may involve waiting for the youngster to hit puberty, a time when tics will often go into remission by themselves. Sometimes the "wait it out" treatment involves just waiting (rather than waiting for a particular age or stage) because tics can disappear shortly after they first appear, no matter the age of the sufferer. In a couple of months or more, many children and teens who experience tics will have a full remission without any treatment. In these quick on-off cases, the tics tend to be mild and don't cause significant interference with happiness or functioning. Therefore, the doctor is right: nothing needs to be done apart from waiting.

When tics are caused by PANDAS, proper antibiotic treatment for the streptococcal infection may bring about a remission of neuropsychiatric symptoms. When it doesn't, the standard treatments for Tic Disorders (including the "wait" strategy described above) can be administered.

The "Stress-Reduction" Approach

Sometimes, however, waiting doesn't yield the desired result. Year after year, the tics persist. Over time, tics may change their form and their severity, one tic replacing another or sometimes, new tics co-existing with old ones. It becomes more important to reduce the frequency and intensity of such tics in order to prevent psychosocial, academic or work-related difficulties.

A treatment that may sometimes be recommended by professionals for these persistent tics is stress reduction. It has been noted that tics increase as stress increases and therefore reducing stress can help reduce tics. We should be clear here that stress does not *cause* tics. Rather, it may *trigger* tics in a brain that is biologically sensitive to the tic dynamic and it can also aggravate tics that are already present, just as all other aspects of our physical and mental health are aggravated by stress. This means that our headaches, backaches, pain syndromes, digestive problems, skin conditions, fibromyalgia, sleeping issues, anxiety symptoms, depressed moods, addictions, mental health symptoms AND our tics all increase when our stress is higher. And all of our physical and mental symptoms tend to improve when we incorporate stress reduction strategies into our life. These include, but are not limited to the following practices:

- Improving life/work balance, reducing pressure, modifying daily demands

- Learning and using daily relaxation techniques such as meditation, self-hypnosis, autogenic relaxation strategies, breathwork or yoga (many of these can be app-assisted these days)

- Improving our total social support system as well as nurturing friendships and meeting with others who have similar issues (in this case, a Tic Disorder)

- Doing regular exercise

- Adding creativity, spirituality and fun to the weekly schedule

- Receiving psychotherapy, counseling and/or biofeedback training

Self-care and stress reduction never hurts anyone and almost always helps in some way, but of course it isn't always enough to eradicate our more intense mental and physical health conditions. When, despite using stress reduction strategies, tics are still problematic, there are other more aggressive interventions that can be called upon.

The "Behavioral" Approach

The first professional level of intervention usually recommended for tics is some form of behavior therapy. There are 3 main types of behavior therapy that have been studied: Habit Reversal Therapy (HRT), Comprehensive Behavioral Intervention for Tics (CBIT) and Exposure and Response Prevention (ERP). Each of these therapies helps sufferers become more conscious of their tic behavior and more in control of the course it will take. People are taught to become aware of pre-tic sensations, helped to find strategies for tolerating those sensations, and helped to choose competing (more socially appropriate) responses so that the tic itself is replaced with a different action. This can help a person of any age do better (and feel better) in social, academic, professional, familial and other interpersonal settings. Each treatment varies in the details of the approach but all are forms of behavioral modification.

None of the behavior therapies cure Tic Disorders or even eradicate tics, but they do provide strategies to help minimize the *disruptive effects* of tics in one's life. Although currently considered the front-line treatment for mild and moderate tics, behavior therapy is still a limited intervention. Current researchers point to the need for the development of treatments that will provide far greater relief for tic sufferers.

Meanwhile, it is very important and valuable to reduce the negative life consequences of disruptive tics. Pediatricians and general practitioners can refer patients to specially trained practitioners who practice one of the behavioral therapies. There are also self-help materials available in book form, online courses and medical apps. These are especially appropriate for those suffering from mild to moderate tic disorders. The preferred treatment for persistent and complex tics will usually be in-person behavior therapy, especially CBIT.

The "Medical" Approach

There are people who do not experience sufficient respite from tics even after making stress-reducing lifestyle adjustments and trying behavior therapy. When tics are having a major negative impact on one's life, the use of medication will often be recommended. Unfortunately, at the moment there is no medical cure for tics. However, some medications have been found to lessen their severity. For instance, dopamine blockers such as fluphenazine, haloperidol (Haldol), risperidone (Risperdal) and pimozide (Orap) are being prescribed to help control tics. Like many antipsychotic drugs, these medicines can produce unpleasant side effects such as weight gain, and ironically, involuntary repetitive movements, as well as other symptoms. Tetrabenazine (Xenazine) is also used in the treatment of tic disorders, and it too can sometimes produce a number of uncomfortable side-effects, including depression. Because of the side-effect profile of these medications, they are understandably usually reserved for those times when a Tic disorder manifests in severe and life-impacting symptoms.

Other drugs and treatments currently used in the treatment of tic disorders and accompanying conditions include anti-depressant and anti-anxiety medications, psychotherapy, and - experimentally at this time - deep brain stimulation. While some of these interventions are aimed directly at tics, others are directed more at the "accompanying conditions" than at the tics themselves. We will learn more about this below. Psychotherapy, for example, can help a person deal with the negative effects that tics might have on self-concept, interpersonal relationships, and academic and professional performance, while it is less likely to directly affect the tic condition itself except by way of stress reduction.

The "Complementary and Alternative Treatment" (CAM) Approach

Many forms of integrative medicine (also known as alternative medicine or complementary and alternative medicine) have been employed in the treatment of Tic Disorders. There are insufficient research studies to affirm the efficacy of these interventions, but individuals who haven't found sufficient relief from their tics, or those who are concerned about the side-effects of medicinal treatment, often turn to treatments outside of the traditional psychological and medical realms. You can read about their experiences online. The following interventions have been used or are being studied for the treatment of Tic Disorders:

- Biofeedback
- Music therapy
- Herbal medicine
- Chinese medicine
- Chiropractic treatment
- Massage therapy and/or bodywork
- Nutritional therapy
- Ayurvedic medicine
- Cannabis
- Homeopathy
- Nutraceutical Therapy (use of vitamins and minerals)
- Hypnotherapy

Consulting a licensed naturopath or CAM practitioner with experience and success in treating tics will usually be the safest way to approach "natural" treatments, since these treatments can produce side-effects and/or interact with a person's health conditions or other medicines and treatments they are receiving.

Another interesting alternative approach to the treatment of tics involves the investigation of TRIGGERS. Some people have found that their tics emerge or are aggravated in the presence of environmental triggers such as any of the following:

- Foods and beverages

- Medications

- Sounds, perfumes and other sensory elements

- Toxins

- Weather conditions

The trigger-search concept is similar to the process found in other health conditions such as migraine or asthma. It seems that people who are sensitive to environmental stimuli are vulnerable to experiencing certain physical symptoms. Those interested in this approach to working with tics should search out a practitioner who works with the Trigger theory. A popular self-help resource for this protocol is the book "Tourette Syndrome: Stop Your Tics by Learning What Triggers Them" by Sheila Rogers DeMare. Sheila has also written a book that explores alternative tic treatments in detail ("Natural Treatments for Tics and Tourette's").

CHAPTER THREE
THE BFTT APPROACH

The purpose of this book is to introduce you to one more possible treatment for Tic Disorders, one that I've seen tremendous success with over the past three decades but one that you've almost certainly never heard of. It is called BFTT, an acronym for "Bach Flower Therapy for Tics."

Bach Flower Therapy is the use of Bach Flower Remedies to help address emotional and physical symptoms. BFTT is the use of Bach Flower Remedies to specifically treat tics (see section below, "What are Bach Flower Remedies?" to learn about the flower essences and how they help). BFTT helps people who are suffering with mild, moderate and severe tics, whether those tics have been around for only a short time or for decades. When BFTT works, there is no need to use any other treatment - no need to search for and remove environmental triggers, no need to manage tic behaviors with arduous, time-consuming and sometimes costly behavioral therapy and no need to take strong medications that can produce unpleasant side-effects. Most importantly, when this treatment works, it puts an end to tics! Therefore, because it is inexpensive, painless, safe, side-effect free and easier than all of the other currently available tic treatment options, you might think of BFTT as a FIRST intervention for any tic condition. If it doesn't work (and there is *no* treatment that works for everyone all the time), the traditional evidence-based medical treatments and/or CAM options described above are always available to explore next.

Because I have personally witnessed the enduring and profound improvement that BFTT has almost always brought about in tic sufferers, I want to share this intervention with you. I want YOU to have the opportunity to experience this relief yourself. I don't sell Bach Flower Remedies - you can purchase them in any health food store and online. My profit will be the happiness gained from knowing I've helped someone attain greater peace and joy in living a tic-free life. Relief from tics is important for everyone, but especially for children whose still fragile sense of self is particularly threatened by the odd-looking, mockable behaviors that tics can sometimes produce. Reducing and eliminating tics is transformative.

If It's So Great, Why Haven't I Heard of Yet?

As I mentioned, few people know that this treatment option for tics exists. Your doctor has probably never heard of it (and might laugh out loud if you share it). Your naturopath, although almost certainly familiar with Bach Flower Therapy, probably isn't aware that the remedies can profoundly help tics. Even professional Bach Flower Therapists may have never used the remedies to treat a Tic Disorder. Since people don't know about it and because it is not a drug that pharmaceutical companies want to research in order to market (Bach Flower Remedies are already available in stores and online around the world), there is no research on the efficacy of Bach Flower Therapy for the treatment of tics. Even research on the efficacy of Bach Flower Remedies for other problems (such as stress or anxiety) is exceedingly sparse and consists mostly of poorly designed and insufficiently populated studies that routinely report no significant therapeutic effect.

If you are the "scientific type" by profession, family background and/ or temperament, you may outright reject any form of non-evidence based alternative treatment, in which case you will naturally opt for the behavioral or medicinal therapies described earlier for the treatment of your (or your loved one's) tics.

However, for those of you who have had some success in your life with an alternative treatment or are just curious and open-minded by nature, or if you are absolutely desperate to subdue your disturbing tics and have had no luck with any other approach or no desire to try something medicinal, please continue reading to find out why a trial of BFTT may be the ticket to success.

What are Bach Flower Remedies?

Even if you have never heard of Bach Flower Therapy or Bach Flower Remedies, you likely suspect that they have something to do with flowers! Indeed, Bach Flowers are healing remedies derived from various plants. Today, they are often referred to as "flower essences" rather than "flower remedies" but the terms both refer to the same small one-ounce bottles of therapeutic water. You probably already know that the healing properties of plants have been harnessed since ancient times. For example, medicinal herbs (botanicals) involve the use of flowers, leaves, seeds, roots, stems and bark of plants in human and animal healing. Homeopathy is another healing modality that often employs herbs but prepares them differently from herbal tinctures. You may have heard of aromatherapy - essential oils also derived from seeds, leaves, roots, stems, petals and the bark of various plants. And of course, healing plants have inspired the preparation of many of our "regular medicines" as well.

Bach Flower Remedies are prepared with water and the flowering part of a plant, but the final product actually contains only the water (the essence) and no plant parts at all. The full method of preparation will be described below.

Note: While some of you are learning about Bach Flowers for the first time, many people around the world are familiar with the popular Bach Flower product called "Rescue Remedy." Rescue Remedy is a preparation made from five remedies in the Bach healing system and is used to calm the fight-or-flight (panic) response in humans and animals. What you may not know is that Rescue Remedy is actually part of a larger system of 38 Flower Remedies developed almost 100 years by Dr. Edward Bach, a British internist. For almost a century, these flowering plants have been used to lift moods, cope with loss, quiet thoughts, reduce irritation and anger, calm anxiety, improve confidence, and more.

How and why do Bach Flowers work? We'll examine some theories shortly. For now, I'll just tell you that I knew about Bach Flowers ever since I was in my early twenties, but I didn't "believe" in them. I was a complete skeptic before I found a reason to change my outlook. Till then, I was of the opinion that people who used this flower-water remedy were either very gullible or just desperate. And then, I joined the desperate group myself.

CHAPTER FOUR

HEALING CAN HAPPEN IN STRANGE WAYS

Decades ago, one of my children developed a severe phobia of robbers and kidnappers. This is a common fear in preschoolers and I didn't think much of it - until it completely overtook our lives. At first, my son just had trouble going to bed at night because of his fear. Later, the fear would start right after dinner. Then it came on before dinner, then in the daytime and eventually it was there from the moment he woke up in the morning till the moment he tearfully and stressfully went to sleep each night. I was a professional mental health practitioner at the time and I had already learned many psychological tools - and I used ALL OF THEM on him. All to no avail.

Two painful years into the problem, I put him on a waiting list to see a child psychiatrist for his by-now debilitating anxiety. One day during this long waiting period, a memory popped into my head. It was a memory of a "natural" treatment for anxiety that a friend had told me about many years earlier - the Bach Flower Remedies.

I had already tried every available non-medical intervention for my little boy's fear, every kind of "evidence-based strategy" and every kind of placebo - everything that I could think of. Nothing was working. I don't recall what triggered the memory of Bach Flower Remedies that particular day but I decided to give them a try. The medical appointment wasn't going to happen anytime soon and we were all still suffering on a daily basis. What did I have to lose?

I knew very little about Bach Flower Remedies at that time. I headed over to a local health food store and found the miniature bottles sitting on a shelf. Beside them was a small pamphlet that described the 38 different remedies, what they were used for and how to take them. One of the remedies was specifically recommended for fears such as the fear of robbers. Perfect! I bought it and gave it to my son that night - two drops from the dropper in a bit of water, as the pamphlet described. Still, I didn't hold any great expectations.

The next morning, my son woke up, and for the first time in more than two years, he was "normal." He didn't start the day off wondering where the robbers were as he had been doing for so long. He just got up and played as if there was never an issue with robbers, as if the whole thing simply didn't exist. I couldn't believe it, but I was still unsure where this was going. Were we just enjoying a few minutes of reprieve? The day went on and there was not a single mention of robbers. Same for the next day and the day after that and forever more - my son had experienced a one-dose cure for his fear of robbers. I was incredulous and curious. Was this a grand coincidence - just the odd timing of administering this remedy and the expiration date of his fear? Or could it actually be that this innocuous-looking bottle of water actually *did* something? I had no idea, but I wanted to learn more. (By the way, the psychiatrist never did end up calling us to schedule that long awaited appointment, and because we didn't need it anymore anyway, my child was spared the possibly of receiving powerful, brain altering medication at such a tender age.)

Frankly, I was blown away. Having been stunned by what looked like a powerful effect of the flower remedy, I considered for the first time that there may be a real place in the world of emotional healing for the Bach Flower Remedies. I decided to undertake professional certification in Bach Flower Therapy from the British Institute of Homeopathy. My instructor was a registered psychologist as well as a homeopath and Bach Flower Practitioner. When I took the course I wasn't sure what I would do with the knowledge. I just knew that I wanted to know more.

All About Bach Flowers

The first thing I learned was how Bach Flower Remedies are made and used. Unfortunately, that initial information only left me feeling more uncertain and confused. Dr. Bach could apparently feel "energies" and would select a plant to be included in his healing system based on information that he "intuited." I didn't relate to or understand these concepts.

Having selected a plant for its healing powers, Dr. Bach would then take its flower, place it in water for a few hours - in sunlight or over a heat source - then discard the flower and keep the water. He would then bottle the water and add some brandy to it to protect the essence against germs and bacteria growing within the bottle. This mixture of water with brandy was known as "the mother tincture." The mother tincture would be further diluted by placing two drops of it into one ounce of water. This was then sold as a stock bottle - the small remedy bottle found on store shelves and online. For self-help treatment, one places two drops from the stock bottle in up to 8 oz. of water or other liquid, and drinks it. That's the treatment.

I had a lot of trouble processing this information because it simply didn't fit into my world view. However, while taking the certification course, I was exposed to a new way of thinking. In this new perspective, in addition to the existence of cognitive neural networks that generate thoughts and influence feelings, and in addition to physical processes that affect emotions and behaviors, there is another whole system of internal influence: the human energy system. This is the system utilized by healers who practice acupuncture, acupressure, yoga, qigong, chakra healing, Reiki, Touch for Health, energy psychology and many other modalities. Although many of these interventions had been around for thousands of years, I was only just becoming aware of the theories underlying their utility. For me, these were radical concepts outside my own frame of reference. So I decided to apply my own frame of reference derived from my traditional psychological education: from that perspective I tried to answer the question "Why might flower remedies facilitate healing?" I came up with a few possible explanations.

#1: Bach Flower Remedies work due to the placebo effect.

The Oxford Dictionary defines the placebo effect as a "beneficial effect produced by a placebo drug or treatment, which cannot be attributed to the properties of the placebo itself, and must therefore be due to the patient's belief in that treatment." In other words, people heal despite the fact that the placebo drug or treatment they received contained no healing properties. Indeed, countless studies demonstrate that what people *think* can affect their personal health. The healing results of placebos are not imaginary; they are very real. But they are *brought about* by human imagination. In other words, if people THINK that a treatment has the power to cure, they may be cured by it even if that treatment has no intrinsic healing properties.

What's even more fascinating is that research shows that a placebo can heal even when a person KNOWS that it is a placebo! Since feeling better - often at long last - is the goal, most people don't mind being cured by a "mere placebo" - they are more than happy to move on if it cures their cancer or excruciating knee pain.

It might be possible then, that Bach Flower Remedies heal because of the placebo effect: people hope and expect them to heal and so they do! (By the way, recent research indicates that even psychotropic medications like antidepressants may be exerting their beneficial impact on mild and moderate cases of depression primarily because of the placebo effect!) My only question about this theory is that when it comes to Bach Flower Remedies, many people DON'T expect them to "work" and they still do. Also, they work on plants, animals and infants, all of whom are not subject to the "placebo effect." I still had questions.

#2: Bach Flowers heal medical and psychological conditions by treating underlying emotional stress.

This was the viewpoint advanced by Dr. Bach himself, a medical physician who used the remedies to treat his patients' medical issues. According to his understanding of the body-mind connection (a concept widely accepted today), the remedies facilitate physical healing by releasing and healing deep emotional stress. Once stress is relieved, the body can heal itself. Applied to the world of tics, if the recent wave of TikTok Tics was indeed triggered by COVID-19 restrictions (the coronavirus), Bach Flowers could help the tics go into remission by healing the stresses of the past couple of years. Similarly, given that the "neurological tics" - provisional tics, chronic tics and Tourette's - are exacerbated by negative emotional states, lifting emotional stress could free up energy for physical brain healing to occur. In other words, stress relief may be the channel through which these remedies promote the remission of tics. I was open to that explanation!

#3: Things Work Even When We Don't Know Why Yet

Since the late 1980's psychological practitioners have employed a very powerful healing tool called "Emotional Freedom Technique," a type of Energy Psychology. There is indisputable scientific evidence that EFT effectively treats severe trauma symptoms, as well as depression, anxiety and other psychological problems. It was used clinically decades before the American Psychological Association and other professional mental health associations around the world listed it as an official "evidence-based intervention." Nonetheless, there is no mainstream explanation for why it works. Like Bach Flower Remedies, EFT is thought by its developers to utilize the human energy system (in this case, the meridian system). Perhaps the two treatment modalities share common underlying mechanisms that none of us fully understand at this time.

If you think about it, there are countless examples of things we do or use without knowing why or how they work. Take a simple light switch. You may not know the underlying mechanical and electrical principles responsible for the workings of your light switch. However, as long as flicking that little button on your wall causes the room to light up, you'll probably keep flicking it. You don't need to understand what makes it work in order to benefit from it. So until definitive science explains the underlying mechanics of Bach Flower Remedies, we might say that the "proof is in the pudding." The clinical evidence of clients who successfully use BFTT to treat their tic condition may be the best and strongest indicator of all.

CHAPTER FIVE

MY JOURNEY INTO BFTT

A strange thing happened shortly after completing the Bach Flower Training Course.

I received a call from a couple who had heard that I knew something about the Bach Flower Remedies. They asked me to use the remedies to treat their child who had a severe and untreatable (they had already tried everything medically available) tic disorder. At the time, I knew that Bach Flower remedies were used to help improve one's psychological state of mind by calming panic and anxiety, lifting mood, soothing trauma, reducing anger and easing irritability. Tic Disorders were not on my horizon.

In fact, in my practice as a counseling psychologist, helping people with their parenting, marriage and personal stress issues, I did not treat people's ADHD, learning disabilities, seizures or other neurological symptoms. I told the parents that I knew very little about tics, had certainly never treated them with Bach Flower Remedies and couldn't guarantee any results if they decided to try this approach. But given that the remedies were harmless and inexpensive, I said I was willing to help them give it a try if they wanted to - and they definitely did!

I began by asking some questions about their child's personality, behavior and mood, and based on that, designed a treatment bottle for them. They called back a few days later to say that their son's tics had completely subsided on the first day of treatment. Subsequent annual follow-ups over a couple of decades showed that this little fellow's tics never returned. Since meeting with these parents thirty years ago, I would relate their experience to others who happened to mention that they or their child suffered with tics. Many of these people were enthusiastic about conducting their own Bach experiments.

Remarkably, over time, I saw that almost all of the children and adults who tried the Bach remedies for their tics had wonderful results: their tics just went away. Soon it became common for me to receive calls from friends and relatives of the "experimenters" who saw the results for themselves. They, too, wanted to know how to conduct a Bach Flower experiment for themselves or their child who suffered from tics.

Over time, I learned that there were different patterns to the recovery process. I quickly learned that "Day One" cures were actually very rare, although most people experienced dramatic improvement quickly - within days or weeks. Some people only had to take the remedy for a few days before the tics stopped and never returned. Others would take it for some weeks or some months, watching their tics gradually and permanently disappear over that period. The most common pattern I saw was that the tics disappeared - whether after days, weeks or months - and then after some period of time, would return. In these cases, the person would begin treatment again each time the tics returned. This off-on pattern might repeat over the course of a few months or even a couple of years. In these off-on cases, the tics would respond faster and faster on each round of treatment (i.e. requiring only a couple of days of BFTT to induce complete remission) and the remission period between treatments would get longer and longer - stretching from weeks, to a few months and then to many months or a couple of years, and then finally stopping.

I want to emphasize that the most common pattern was that positive results manifested quickly and dramatically. Because tics come and go anyways (the infamous "wax and wane" pattern), one might think that the remedy had nothing to do with the recovery; we know that tics have a tendency to act up and calm down and then disappear without any treatment at all. However for these sufferers, that typical pattern had NOT happened in their lives. They had waited weeks, months, years or decades without any form of serious remission. Yet when they tried BFTT, real remission occurred for the first time. Yes, this could be a coincidence in each case, but the statistical likelihood of that being the explanation is very low.

Of course, there were also a few who found no benefit from the remedies, something that happens with virtually every treatment modality for every mental and physical issue. However, this tended to be a rare exception in the sample of people I had encountered. In addition, there was one person (in my 30 years of watching people's experiments) who reported an unwanted side effect (faintness). Nonetheless, while the available research on the Bach remedies consists of few and small studies, none bear evidence of negative consequences. Here's a quote from WebMd: "Small studies of Bach Flower Remedies have not identified safety concerns."

What we know for certain is that the remedies have been in use around the world for over a century. Obviously many people find them helpful in some way. Now, many more might find them helpful for their tics.

CHAPTER SIX
PREPARATION FOR BFTT

If you are ready to begin a trial of BFTT, we will look at how to select Bach Flower Remedies to treat tics. Each person who uses BFTT will have an individualized treatment bottle - a bottle that contains remedies unique to them. Two family members who are treating their tics will have two different treatment bottles. As mentioned, there are 38 Bach Flower Remedies. Each person selects between one and seven of the remedies for their personalized treatment (or a parent selects the remedies for their child).

Dr. Bach intended that the selection process should be simple enough for a successful *self-help* protocol. As the remedies are broad-acting, making a "wrong" selection isn't something you need to worry about. Whatever you choose will be good enough to get results as long as a couple of the descriptive words for the remedy fits the personality being treated. For example, if a child has a temper, you might choose the remedy called Impatiens which treats irritability and the tendency to be "quick to snap" or you might select Holly which is for the person who gets angry when feeling disrespected or insulted. You can choose both if you haven't exceeded your limit of seven remedies, but if you can only select one because you already have six others selected, then whichever of the two you choose is fine because they are *broad-acting*. This means that both Impatiens and Holly will treat the overall tendency to feel angry.

Some people like to consult a professional Bach Flower Practitioner. If you decide to do this, ask the practitioner to ensure that the remedy Agrimony is included in the treatment bottles (as explained in more detail below). Remember that professional Bach Flower Practitioners (those with recognized training and certification) may or may not have treated tic disorders. They will certainly not be familiar with the term BFTT and they are probably not familiar with the necessity of including Agrimony when addressing a tic disorder. However, they WILL have a very good grasp of the characteristics of the remedies and an excellent knowledge of which ones will be most appropriate for you or your child. This skill will help them create a treatment bottle that should, with the addition of Agrimony, hit the spot.

Having said this, I want to be clear that you definitely DO NOT NEED professional assistance in order to create an effective treatment bottle. Bach Flower Therapy was intended from its inception to be a self-help healing modality. The system is designed to work for YOU - the regular, untrained user.

If you shop for the Bach Flower Remedies in a store, you're likely to find a small brochure near the shelf where the remedies are situated (just as I did all those years ago). The brochure contains a description of each of the remedies - typically one or two sentences long. It is sufficient for users to decide whether a particular remedy is suitable for themselves or their loved one. It is also easy to find descriptions for the flower remedies online. Below, I'll give you my own description for each remedy from which you can select one to six remedies PLUS Agrimony to help you or your loved one with tics. Once you have selected the appropriate remedies, you'll proceed to Chapter Seven where you will find instructions for how to prepare and take them.

When selecting a remedy for yourself or a loved one, consider the areas of personality that could use a bit of help. The remedies are described in terms of the problems that they help address. If a remedy sounds like it's describing an issue that you or your loved one has, put a little check mark beside it. Don't worry if you end up with more than seven check marks altogether - I'll tell you what to do about that later. Also note that the first remedy in the following list (Agrimony) will always automatically be checked off because this remedy must be included when tics are the focus of treatment.

Only select those remedies that describe a personality *tendency* - all of us have experienced each of these states on occasion. We are looking here for a recurring tendency so that the description seems to be portraying a character trait of the person in question. It's also fine if none of these remedy profiles really fit. In that case, Agrimony will be the only remedy applied in the tic treatment.

Ready? Let's begin! Check off each relevant remedy:

☐ *Agrimony:* PUT A CHECK MARK HERE BECAUSE AGRIMONY IS ALWAYS INCLUDED WHEN TREATING TICS. For your information (i.e. in case you eventually want to use Bach Flowers to target a condition other than tics), I will include Agrimony's profile here. Agrimony is helpful for people who have inner tension but outwardly show a happy face. They tend to be peace-lovers who are distressed by and therefore avoid conflict. Inner stress may be expressed by restlessness, disturbed sleep, physical pain or bodily symptoms such as tight muscles, stomach problems, rashes, and frequent mild illnesses. Those who turn to drugs, alcohol or other addictive substances or habits to soothe inner tension, may find that Agrimony reduces their need to do so by helping them recognize, tolerate and release their feelings directly. Since Agrimony exposes suppressed feelings, a person may become uncharacteristically "not so nice" (i.e. irritable, angry, vocal, uncooperative) for a short while after starting this remedy. Although temporarily unpleasant for loved ones, it's a good sign that the feelings have become unblocked and are in the process of releasing.

☐ *Aspen:* For those who have vague fears and dread that "something bad will happen." Aspen is great for children who are afraid of monsters, ghosts and the dark. It helps adults who, for no explicable reason, "have a bad feeling" that some sort of unpreventable catastrophe, harm or even death will occur. Aspen is indicated for a person who suffers with numerous worries, one with or without a formal diagnosis of Generalized Anxiety Disorder (GAD), or who suffers with the chronic feeling that disaster lurks around every corner.

☐ **Beech**: For the person who tends to be judgmental, intolerant, perfectionistic and/or chronically negative. The negativity may be directed inward toward the person himself or outward toward others or toward situations and life in general. Beech is helpful for those who see others as flawed, too slow, too careless, too unintelligent, too boring or otherwise generally deficient. The parent who is highly critical of a particular child or the child for whom nothing is exciting, fun or tasty enough, will tend to see more of the good when taking Beech. Critical, grumpy and chronically irritated, the adult or child who needs Beech often ends up being lonely as well, since this type of personality tends to repel others, including family members. Beech is also indicated when a depressed mood comes from a feeling of chronic dissatisfaction. The Beech dynamic is often found in those with ADHD.

☐ *Centaury:* Centaury people give too much; they have trouble setting normal, healthy and protective boundaries. They are often aware of this and may feel bad about it, viewing themselves as victims or as too weak. Fear of being rejected, disliked or reprimanded can cause them to quickly cave. When asked to help out, they'll say "yes" even when "no" makes far more sense. Centaury people are sometimes "rescuers", focusing their efforts on fixing or helping others rather than paying attention to what's needed in their own lives. Often, those who can benefit from Centaury can also benefit from Willow (see below) which is used to address resentment. Those who give too much inevitably notice that the favor is not returned and usually come to feel resentful about this.

☐ *Cerato:* Cerato helps those who don't trust their own intuition. When it comes to making decisions, these people rely on others for advice, validation and approval before taking action. It's not "expert" advice they seek; they simply need someone else to decide for them before they can take the step they want to take. Deep down they know what they want to do but they can't do it without outside approval. Even after doing much research they may have trouble committing to a path for fear that it may be the wrong one (which would be disastrous and intolerable in their mind rather than just unfortunate and annoying as it would be for others).

☐ *Cherry Plum*: Cherry Plum helps those who feel like they are losing - or are about to lose - control. It is ideal for those who feel like they're about to lose their mind - someone who is panicking for example or who is "cracking" under too much pressure. Cherry Plum helps with explosive anger and violent tendencies, emotional overwhelm, panic, fear of physically or emotionally harming oneself or others, fear of urinating inappropriately or otherwise embarrassing oneself in public, fear of vomiting, fear of dying or going crazy and all other "out of control" feelings. Those who have terrifying nightmares, intense and/or frightening sexual impulses and intense cravings, addictive urges and compulsions, can also benefit from the Cherry Plum remedy.

☐ *Chestnut Bud:* This remedy helps those who are on the immature side (think "class clown") as well as those who have trouble paying attention to details, concentrating on boring subjects (like homework or taxes), remembering things, staying focused, employing appropriate caution and learning from experience. Children and teens who benefit from Chestnut Bud often repeat the same misbehaviors over and over despite the educational interventions of their parents and teachers and even law enforcement agencies. Kids who lie, steal or cheat are candidates for this remedy. Chestnut Bud can be helpful for many who are diagnosed (or self-diagnosed) with ADHD symptoms.

☐ *Chicory*: Chicory is helpful for those who give a lot of themselves but have the ulterior motive of wanting abundant love and appreciation in return. Their response to lukewarm enthusiasm or attention might be some version of "after all I've done for you..." People rarely identify their own need for Chicory but others can see it in what they perceive as manipulative tendencies. For instance, Chicory can help the kind of child who "turns on sweetness" and offers to help out so that the parent will buy a desired item or permit a certain privilege. Chicory is also helpful for the parent who shows love by offering too much help or advice (particularly, unsolicited help and advice!) and for anyone who is interfering, controlling or demanding. Since WE don't usually see ourselves in these ways, we can identify our need for chicory by looking at how others respond to us. "I was just trying to help - I don't know why they seemed so annoyed. They could be more grateful!"

☐ *Clematis:* Clematis helps those who are "spacey" - off in their own dreamworld. Whereas Chestnut Bud helps those who are distracted by sights and sounds, the Clematis child or adult is distracted by the inner world of imagination and daydreams. Those who have been traumatized (with or without a diagnosis of Post-Traumatic-Stress-Disorder) often benefit from this remedy because they can get stuck inside their heads with rumination and flashbacks, leaving them far away from the present moment. This affects attention, memory and learning both at work and at school. However, others may have trouble being grounded for different reasons, such as their personality type. Creatives and artsy dreamers may need a call back to the humdrum world where housework or homework needs to be done. Clematis is grounding, improving attention and memory when problems are caused by dwelling more in the future or the past, than in the here-and-now.

☐ *Crab Apple:* Crab Apple is the "cleansing remedy." It can help those people who suffer intensely from feelings of physical inadequacy and ugliness, unable to tolerate the imperfections and small flaws that characterize the normal human body. For example, a person might be exceedingly self-conscious about imperfect teeth, large ears, frizzy or thin hair, occasional blemishes or other irregularities. In teens and adults this can sometimes lead to the desire for, or undertaking of, multiple surgeries and procedures to correct the perceived flaws. Sometimes eating disorders arise out of the same dynamic. This remedy can be part of the healing protocol for those who've received a diagnosis of BBD (Body Dysmorphic Disorder). Similarly, a desire for perfect order and/or cleanliness in the environment may be brought down to more comfortable levels with the help of Crab Apple. Those whose OCD (Obsessive-Compulsive Disorder) leads to a fear of contamination are also good candidates for Crab Apple. They may find that therapy is more productive and easier to undertake while using the remedy. Finally, victims of abuse who feel broken or dirty can also be helped by this remedy. When PTSD arises after sexual assault or other forms of degradation, the help of Crab Apple might be considered.

☐ **Elm:** When someone feels overwhelmed by all that they have to do, elm can help restore a sense of balance and well-being. People who demand too much of themselves or have trouble delegating tasks or doing less - or doing less well - may be helped by Elm as it increases self-compassion and self-acceptance. Anyone who puts self-care and relaxation last on their list, finding themselves stressed, exhausted, anxious and depressed from having too much to do, should really consider helping themselves to Elm. Unfortunately, it often takes a physical illness to stop such people in their tracks. Even then it's not too late to reach for balance with the help of Elm.

☐ **Gentian:** Gentian helps those who are quickly discouraged after minor setbacks. At the first struggle or difficulty, they'll throw their hands in the air, saying things like "Why bother trying? I won't get picked anyway....it won't work anyway....I can't do it" and so on. Their pessimism causes them to give up way too soon, whether the issue is schoolwork, relationships, an exercise program or whatever. Low frustration tolerance holds them back from success that might otherwise have been attained. Gentian is also a good remedy for those who tend to be pessimistic in general or who suffer from a chronic low-grade depression (previously called "Dysthymia," now known as Persistent Depressive Disorder). It helps to return feelings of confidence and optimism and the resultant willingness to continue trying.

☐ **Gorse:** Gorse renews hope and energy in those who have become depressed as a result of severe disappointment, failure, loss or suffering. Such people have actually tried their best for a long time, invested heavily, and given it their all - but have failed to see success or have lost a great deal. As a result, they have moved beyond the discouragement of the Gentian state to the hopelessness of the Gorse state. Although both Gorse and Mustard (see below) address deep, dark moods, Gorse is indicated when there is a clear REASON for the depressed feelings, whereas Mustard addresses low moods that are biologically triggered. Similarly, although both Gorse and Sweet Chestnut (see below) address feelings of despair, Gorse applies to practical losses whereas Sweet Chestnut addresses existential angst. And finally, although both Gorse and Star of Bethlehem address loss, Gorse addresses the sadness of practical loss while Star of Bethlehem addresses trauma, heartbreak and grief.

☐ *Heather:* There are some people who talk and talk and talk, whether their listener wants to continue listening or not! Heather can help this sort of person come to see that others have needs as well. The "talking syndrome" is often seen in those who have ADHD but it can occur in others as well. In addition, those who need a lot of attention or a lot of possessions, whom others would describe as "a bottomless pit" or insatiable, are also candidates for Heather. "Drama queens/kings" (excitable, needy, demanding) and highly emotional people also benefit from this remedy. Parents will find it easy to identify Heather as the remedy that can help a very demanding child but, as was the case for Chicory, we adults are unlikely to see *ourselves* in the Heather dynamic. We might guess that it could be helpful if we find that people rarely give us the time or attention we'd like or feel that we deserve.

☐ *Holly:* Holly can help those who are frequently angry, hostile, defensive, jealous, spiteful and/or paranoid (suspicious). Underlying these emotions is insecurity and low self-esteem and a corresponding strong need to feel loved and valued. Holly people are sensitive and easily insulted or offended, but instead of showing their hurt, they show anger. When attacked, they counter-attack instead of sharing their hurt and vulnerability. Holly can help those who are highly competitive and those who feel hateful toward others - a common dynamic that occurs between siblings. Again, we adults may not identify with the characteristics treated by Holly. We will more easily see it as a resource when we frequently feel misunderstood, unfairly blamed, attacked or disrespected and when we feel surrounded by uncaring and untrustworthy people.

☐ *Honeysuckle:* Honeysuckle helps those who suffer from homesickness or who are stuck in the past, remembering (and favoring) "the good ol' days." It can help older people who tend to dwell on their past with nostalgia rather than focusing on, and investing in, a positive present and future. It also helps people who have been separated from loved ones through death, divorce, moving, travelling and so on, and who are now consumed with loneliness or grief (when the primary emotion is "missing" then Honeysuckle is the most helpful remedy, whereas when the primary emotion is grieving, then Star of Bethlehem is most indicated. However, both can be taken at the same time). Changes such as retiring, going to sleepover camp or away for schooling, can also provoke the Honeysuckle state. Children who act younger than their chronological age - sucking their thumb, struggling with toilet training past toddlerhood, walking around with a pacifier and so on - can be thought of as having trouble moving on and therefore would also be candidates for Honeysuckle. Ditto for middle-aged or older people who dress or act decades younger.

☐ *Hornbeam:* Hornbeam helps those with boredom and tendencies to procrastinate, as well as those who are unenthused or listless. The remedy is particularly suited to those who delay getting started on tasks but then once immersed in them, wake up and do quite well. Hornbeam helps instill both energy and a brighter mood.

☐ *Impatiens*: An impatient attitude is helped by the Remedy called Impatiens! Some people can't tolerate slow, methodical movement; they move and talk quickly, rushing everything along. Slow traffic and lineups are intolerable for them. Impatiens also helps those who are easily irritated and quick to explode in anger as well as those who feel like they are "wired," running on nervous energy or "close to the edge." Impatiens is a remedy that is often useful for those diagnosed with ADHD.

☐ *Larch:* Larch helps people who lack self-confidence and/or fear failure when faced with performance situations such as auditions, examinations, interviews and other situations where competition is the critical element. People who need Larch are typically capable but think others are probably more so. They lack belief in themselves even though they are competent and successful. An A student who fears failure at every exam would be a good candidate for Larch.

☐ *Mimulus*: Mimulus is very useful for those with specific fears and phobias, such as fears of kidnappers, spiders, lightning, dogs, needles, bees and so on. (Mimulus helps *prevent* fears but the remedy Rock Rose will be helpful in addressing a fear that has already been provoked (i.e. take Mimulus when worrying about giving a presentation and take Rock Rose when feeling panic at the time of the presentation) Those who suffer from health anxiety often benefit tremendously from Mimulus. Also, people who worry about a lot of different things or who are generally nervous will find Mimulus helpful. Mimulus helps the symptoms we typically see in Anxiety Disorders when the anxiety can be named (i.e. worrying about finances, health or dying; being phobic of flying, driving on highways, water, or bugs; worrying about being fired or contracting diseases or feeling shy around strangers). Fears that can't be specifically named ("I'm afraid something bad will happen") are better treated by Aspen (see above).

☐ *Mustard:* Mustard is helpful for "dark cloud" depressed moods that come out of nowhere and for no particular reason. One's own genetic constitution can create a depressive reaction to hormones (such as occur in menstrual cycles, childbirth and menopause) or to grey skies, food, environmental factors, and other natural conditions, as well as to one's own thoughts. Mustard can help when there is a profound lack of joy, energy, enthusiasm and motivation. Mustard helps lift the gloomy, dark, unhappy and listless mindset characteristic of these depressed states. Note that when the main cause of a depressed mood is negativity, discouragement, grief, overwhelm and so on, other remedies may be more appropriate.

☐ *Oak:* The Oak person is a very hard worker with a great sense of responsibility to do what is right or necessary no matter how hard or exhausting that will be. This person plows on, ignoring bodily cues of fatigue and burnout, often till the point of mental or physical collapse (or both). "Oak types" who are students tend to push themselves too hard, failing to give themselves appropriate breaks and downtime. Oak helps a person find balance again, increasing motivation for self-care and activities that bring personal joy.

☐ **Olive:** Olive helps revive those suffering from spiritual, physical, mental and emotional burnout. Olive aids a state of total depletion, like that caused by the Oak dynamic, but not limited to the stress of carrying excessive burdens or overworking. Struggling with a long illness or chronic money problems, raising an impossibly difficult child without adequate support or reprieve, giving unremitting care to an elderly or unwell loved one, going through a lengthy, highly contested divorce or other legal battle, fighting to survive in times of war or other natural disasters, coping with endless business difficulties - enduring any situation that depletes one's reserves on every level, can provoke a need for the help of Olive.

☐ **Pine:** Pine helps low self-esteem, feelings of inadequacy, shame, unworthiness and excessive or unnecessary guilt. It can be used for those who apologize excessively or whose perfectionism causes them to feel incompetent or intrinsically flawed. Whereas Larch helps those who feel like they don't measure up *compared to others,* Pine helps those who don't measure up to their own standards. It eases the relentless torment caused by a powerful inner critic.

☐ **Red Chestnut:** Red Chestnut helps those who worry about the welfare of those closest to them. A child who fears the death of his parents (for no specific reason), a mother who worries excessively about her loved one's problems, or anyone who worries a lot about other people's health, safety or well-being, can benefit from this remedy. When the subject of worry is someone close, choose Red Chestnut. When worried about your own problems, choose Mimulus.

☐ **Rock Rose:** Rock Rose helps ease feelings of panic. Physical symptoms of trauma, such as hypervigilance and the startle response, as well as symptoms of intense anxiety and panic attack, are all helped by Rock Rose. Rock Rose addresses rapid heartbeat, sweaty palms, dizziness, diarrhoea and any of the other mental and bodily symptoms of the fight-or-flight response. Nightmares, shock and terror all respond well to Rock Rose. When your child has a dog phobia and you know you will be in a place that has dogs, bring the Rock Rose along! Similarly bring the Rock Rose if you fear you'll freeze up and not be able to think clearly or perform well during an important interview, exam or presentation. Note that Mimulus would be appropriate to help a child who has a fear of lightning but Rock Rose would be appropriate for that child once he begins to panic because he heard thunder. Taking Mimulus regularly can eventually help "unwire" the phobic response so that it doesn't continue to occur, whereas Rock Rose addresses it when it DOES occur.

☐ **Rock Water**: Rock Water helps people who perfectionistically strive for health, morality, spirituality or some other form of excellence that requires self-denial, self-discipline and restriction. Rock Water helps the person who not only personally maintains these high standards but also strives to get others to adhere to them as well. The Rock Water remedy helps people to "loosen up and let go a little" so that they can both achieve excellence AND enjoy all that life has to offer. Choose Rock Water for your child who refuses to take time off from studying and choose it for yourself when your values prevent you from enjoying relaxation and fun.

☐ **Scleranthus**: Those who have rapidly changing moods (from up to down, or from calm to agitated, for instance) can use Scleranthus to help establish a more even keeled personality. Scleranthus can also help those who have trouble making decisions due to this same inner instability - "Maybe I should do it...no maybe I shouldn't.." Whereas indecisive Cerato folks seek the advice of others in order to resolve their inner conflict, Scleranthus people just fluctuate back and forth in their own minds, endlessly debating the pros and cons of a choice. Scleranthus can also help the scattered, "all-over-the-place" type of person who can't seem to settle on a stable path forward. You might offer Scleranthus to your teen who simply can't decide between two or three equally attractive post-secondary options. If the teen can't think of *any* direction to pursue after high school, then Wild Oat (see below) would be more appropriate.

☐ **Star of Bethlehem**: This remedy treats trauma and shock to the system. A person who has had a life-threatening accident, or witnessed something terrifying or has gone through bullying, abuse or any type of neglect of mistreatment, frequently suffers negative psychological consequences. Those who are dealing with serious illness or invasive surgery, have witnessed the suffering or death of a loved one, have discovered cruel betrayal by a deeply trusted person or have undergone other traumatic experiences, can become deeply unsettled. The result of intense, frightening and disturbing life experiences can be mistrust, fear, hypervigilance, numbing, memory loss, panic attacks, insomnia, nightmares, intrusive thoughts, phobias and more. Whenever someone has experienced a specific or chronic traumatic situation, Star of Bethlehem can provide support and help ease symptoms. Star of Bethlehem is also the remedy to turn to in times of grief.

☐ *Sweet Chestnut:* Profound loss, devastating failure, immovable obstacles, constant setbacks and other sources of intense pain can sometimes throw a person into a state of existential angst, deep despair, even a wish to die. Sweet Chestnut can be called upon in this darkest of emotional places, the "dark night of the soul." Children and teens can find themselves in this place just as adults can, but usually for different reasons. Some 5 year olds express a wish to die - although they aren't suicidal (planning their death). This can happen due to a genetic tendency toward despair and hopelessness, in which case Sweet Chestnut can be helpful in unwinding the inherited trait (always consult a mental health professional when a child of any age expresses hopelessness or despair but you can use Sweet Chestnut along with appropriate intervention or when an "all clear" has been indicated by an appropriate professional assessment). Similarly, don't dismiss teenage angst as "hormonal" - always treat despair seriously and go ahead and offer Sweet Chestnut along with appropriate psychological treatment. When suicidality IS an issue, Sweet Chestnut can help a person WANT to undertake the necessary medical and psychological treatments that will restore wellness. It can be offered even if a person has already been taken for psychiatric treatment against his will.

☐ *Vervain:* This remedy is for people whose passion sometimes gets in their own way. It can help those whose strong sense of justice or unfairness causes them excessive suffering. For instance, Vervain can help the child who is always complaining that things are "unfair", that the sibling has more or better and that they themselves are somehow missing out. The Vervain mind tends to be rigid and Vervain types may sometimes become fanatical about their deeply held beliefs. In some cases, they will strive endlessly to convince others of their principled stance. At times, this produces great achievements and at other times, it only produces difficulty in social relationships. We may not see the Vervain dynamic in ourselves but when feeling extremely frustrated that others "just don't get it," we might consider accessing relief with the help of Vervain. Vervain helps those whose intense drive, enthusiasm or energy keeps them so stressed that their health suffers and/or they are unable to wind down and sleep at night. In addition, Vervain can be helpful for hyperactive children and adults with or without a formal diagnosis of ADHD.

☐ *Vine:* Vine brings perspective and balance to those who are very strong-willed ("my way or the highway"), to people who are bossy, controlling, inflexible, opinionated, pushy and aggressive (sometimes to the point of violence). Vine is often characteristic of those who have ADHD, ODD, OCD and other mental health conditions characterized by rigidity and inflexibility. Again, this is an easy dynamic to spot in our loved ones and less so in ourselves. We might think of it when we feel that OTHER people are so stubborn! This works because if we want someone to do something (because we are in need of Vine because we're on the bossy, pushy side) and they refuse to do what we want, we tend to call THEM stubborn.

☐ *Walnut:* Walnut eases transition and can be used to help negotiate big and small life changes such as the first day of school, moving homes, going away to camp or school, divorcing, entering puberty, going through childbirth, menopause and so on. Walnut can also help those who are overly affected by things that they see, hear or read - for example, people who are very disturbed by seeing a death scene in a movie (even a children's cartoon film) or by hearing a frightening piece of news or by reading a ghost story.

☐ **Water Violet:** The Water Violet personality is reserved, private, introverted, reflective, intelligent, and often lonely. Loneliness is a by-product of being highly selective in choosing like-minded companions; unfortunately not many people "qualify." Water Violet helps create an openness to others, facilitating access to the pleasures and comforts of more plentiful social relationships.

☐ **White Chestnut:** A "noisy brain" is quieted by White Chestnut. Those who ruminate, obsess and otherwise are bothered by constant or intrusive thoughts and/or images, can find relief with the help of this remedy. It especially benefits those who suffer from insomnia because they "can't turn their brain off." Those who have OCD and especially "Pure O" may find this remedy helpful. Those whose ruminations are caused by trauma can take both Star of Bethlehem and White Chestnut. It can also be paired with Mimulus for those who worry about the issues that concern them. White Chestnut and Scleranthus can help put an end to the endless thinking that is going into a simple decision. White Chestnut and Aspen can address the non-stop worry of "what if something bad happens?" Whenever a person is overthinking, White Chestnut is the indicated remedy.

☐ **Wild Oat:** Wild Oat can help those who struggle to find direction. They have lost touch with their inner guidance that normally propels people to seek a specific path, education, training, profession, business opportunity or other outlet for their skills and abilities. They don't know which road to take; they feel blocked. Wild Oat helps release that block to help them find their way.

☐ **Wild Rose:** This remedy addresses apathy. It helps those who have resigned themselves to an unsatisfactory or unhappy situation or to a less satisfying path, because they lack either the energy or willpower to improve or fight for something better. They feel like there's no point. Those who need Gentian also feel discouraged but only after encountering a setback or failure. Wild Rose helps those who haven't even tried and aren't about to - they assume doing so would be a waste of time or they simply haven't got the necessary strength or vision. "No, I'm not going to College. It'll be too hard."

Wild Rose helps to revitalize vision, hope and determination.

☐ **_Willow:_** Willow helps people who feel resentful and victimized, those who tend to blame others rather than looking at their own role in events. Willow also helps lift the bitterness, depression and negativity that can result from feeling or being chronically wronged. As the Willow state can sometimes be hard to identify in ourselves, we might consider this remedy when we feel the pain of being badly treated.

Okay, add up your checkmarks. At this point, you might have only Agrimony or perhaps you have Agrimony plus several others that you've selected. If you have seven or fewer remedies in total, you are ready to move on to Chapter Seven where you'll learn how to prepare them in a treatment bottle and how to take them on a daily basis.

However, if you've selected more than seven remedies (including Agrimony), you'll need to narrow down your choices. Do this by keeping Agrimony and six other remedies that you feel are the "**most** descriptive" of the person in question. You can keep the discarded remedies in mind for the future because you may decide, as treatment progresses, that some remedies are no longer needed and others can take their place. Or you may find that the discarded remedies are also no longer relevant. When it comes to BFTT, your current selection of remedies may be used indefinitely, or over time, it may make sense to change the selection somewhat. Changes in the remedy bottle are made for either of the following 2 reasons:

1. The remedy isn't working as well as you'd like and you want to see if other remedies might be more helpful

2. A trait that you were treating is no longer apparent. For instance, your original bottle contained Mimulus for separation anxiety, but now, 4 months later, separation anxiety is no longer an issue. When you mix the next bottle, you won't include Mimulus.

Now that you've chosen the remedies you think are the best fit for now, you are ready to learn how to prepare and take them. Let's move on to Chapter Seven.

CHAPTER SEVEN
THE BFTT TREATMENT PROTOCOL

Now that you've selected your remedies, you're ready to prepare a treatment bottle. For this you'll need a one-ounce glass bottle with a glass dropper. You can get this from a bottle distributor, but more conveniently you can get it wherever the Bach Flower Remedies are sold - health food stores, online, on Amazon and elsewhere. Look for a "Bach Mixing Bottle." I always suggest getting two of them so that a second one is ready to prepare as soon as you've emptied (but not yet cleaned) the first botte. I'll explain this shortly.

You'll also need to purchase the remedies you've selected.

Finally, you'll need a bit of unflavored brandy, whiskey or vodka to add as a preservative against bacteria growing in your bottle. Alternatively, you can use vegetable glycerin or apple cider vinegar for this purpose (but be aware that apple cider vinegar will give your remedy a distinctly apple cider vinegar flavor which is not usually appealing).

Once you've assembled your bottle, the remedies, and the preservative, prepare the Treatment Bottle as follows.

1. Fill your glass mixing bottle with plain (not fizzy) water. Any kind will do, including tap water, filtered water or bottled water. You'll notice that your Bach Mixing Bottle (one ounce/30 ml bottle) has sides that go straight up and then curve toward a thinner neck. We'll call that curve "the shoulder" of the bottle. Fill the bottle with your water until the shoulder of the bottle (see photo at the end of this chapter).

2. Now add two drops of each remedy to the bottle. Admittedly, this is a tiny amount, so if more than two drops happen to

fall into the bottle while you are squeezing the dropper, don't worry about it. There is no problem of an "overdose" - you are just wasting a bit of the remedy. Also note that adding more drops will not make the remedy "stronger" or more effective.

3. You'll find that there is a small space left in the bottle now, between the curve and the skinny neck of the bottle. In that space, place about a teaspoon of the unflavored brandy or other chosen preservative.

How to Take the Remedy

Once your bottle is prepared, it is ready for use. At first, effective treatment requires four doses a day - morning, mid-day, afternoon and evening. The frequency of doses diminishes as treatment progresses, as will be explained below. If you are taking the remedy four times a day, your treatment bottle should last 3 ½ - 4 weeks. To take the remedy to treat your tics, follow these simple steps:

1. Place 4 drops (again, don't worry if a bit more comes out of your dropper) in up to 8 ounces of liquid. Examples of suitable liquids are water, milk, juice, tea, coffee, soup...anything non-fizzy. The liquid can be hot or cold. If you aren't thirsty and don't want to drink a whole cup of liquid, no worries: you can put the 4 drops into just a tablespoon of liquid - or into any amount of liquid, up to 8 ounces. This Bach-infused liquid should be consumed some time in the morning, with or without food.

2. Repeat Step 1 above three more times - once around noon, again in the late afternoon, and then one more time in the evening. Exact times aren't important. Just take the remedy four times during the day: in the morning, around mid-day, in the late afternoon and in the evening.

3. After 3 or 4 weeks, you'll have emptied the treatment bottle and can prepare a new one. To do so, wash out the dropper with hot water. Boil the bottle itself in water for 3 minutes or

so. This is to prevent the growth of bacteria and germs in the bottle. Once boiled, the bottle can be filled again with water and your selected remedies.

Every time you start taking a Bach remedy you will start this way - 4 drops, four times a day. This means you will have a total of 16 drops of the remedy daily. However, as you'll see shortly, the frequency of the dose will decrease as your symptoms improve. You won't always be taking it four times a day and there will even be times when you won't be taking it at all. Let's see how this works:

How to Adjust the Remedy

Treatment always starts, as described above, by taking the remedy four times a day. When the tics are decreasing significantly, begin taking the remedy three times a day. When there is even more improvement, move down to two times a day. When the tics are virtually gone, take it once a day - if you remember! When you start forgetting to take it or just don't feel like taking it anymore, then stop taking it. Just use your gut feeling for when to make these changes; if your tics act up you can always up your dose and then lower it again later when they're quieting down. Once you stop taking the remedy completely, you have ended a round of treatment.

After a while, tics may return. There are exceptions - in some people, the first round of treatment will be the last, bringing a complete end to tics. In others, the tics will be back - perhaps triggered by a new personal stress. In this case, start taking the remedy again, consuming it four times a day (the schedule for the beginning of each round of treatment).

Again, as the tics diminish, move down from four times a day, to three times a day, to twice a day, once a day, and then, when mostly forgetting or not caring to take it anymore, stop treatment again. Continue this pattern for the second round, third round, and however many rounds of treatment are required before the tics don't return at all.

During the course of healing, rounds of treatment and periods that are tic-free typically change in length. For instance, let's look at Alex's healing journey: Alex took four months to complete the first round of his treatment, meaning at the end of four months his tics had stopped. All remained well for three months, when some tics came back, so Alex started a new round of BFTT. On this second round, it took only two months to resolve the tics and this time the tics were more mild than in the past. Alex then remained tic-free for six months before some tics showed up. Treatment began again but was necessary for only a few weeks - and the tic-free state lasted 10 months. When a couple of mild tics next appeared, Alex began treatment again, needing only a few days of BFTT before the tics disappeared. This time he stayed in remission for years. Subsequently, Alex would help himself to BFTT for a day or two when he recognized a tic visitor, but eventually even that was no longer necessary.

In summary, treatment proceeds as follows:

1. Take the remedy four times a day - morning, mid-day, afternoon, evening.

2. When symptoms improve significantly, take it three times a day.

3. When tics are almost gone, move down to two times a day.

4. When tics are mostly not happening, take the remedy once a day or so.

5. When you lose the motivation to continue treatment because there are no tics, stop the treatment.

6. If tics return, start taking the remedy four times a day again and then continue steps 2 - 6 until the tics no longer return. The key to success is repeatedly starting rounds of treatment until the tics are completely gone.

A successful treatment with Bach Flower Remedies ENDS at some point. For example, if you are using the remedies to treat your tic disorder, there should come a time when tics simply do not return. When that happens, there is no further need to take the remedy. BFTT is not used to prevent tics; it is used to stop them from occurring.

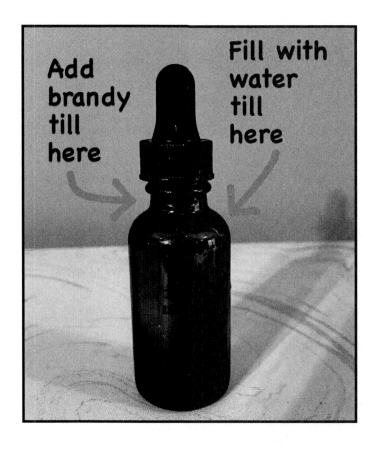

Q & A

How long do Bach Flowers take to work? When will I see improvement?

As explained earlier, usually people experience rapid and significant improvement with BFTT, often within the first days and weeks of treatment. But if that doesn't happen to you or your child, don't give up! Use at least one full treatment bottle - that is about a month's worth of 4 doses a day. If you experience no change whatsoever, but are willing to continue your experiment, then reconsider your selection of remedies. Go through the checklist again and see if you can make changes that might make sense. Continue treatment for a second and third month with that bottle. (making your BFTT trial a total of 3 months). If it's not working at all for you or your child, then I'd say you gave it a fair try. You can continue for as many months as you want to continue trying, but using it for less than 3 months is NOT a fair trial. Sometimes tics occur for quite awhile but in a significantly milder form and then eventually vanish. If you don't mind taking the remedy and you feel that it IS helping at least somewhat, then just continue to take it. Keep in mind that BFTT can be taken at the same time that you are undergoing behavioral therapy for tics if you'd like and you can even continue with it while investigating CAM or medical approaches (as long as your practitioner doesn't object) because Bach Flower Remedies do not interact with other substances.

How do I know when to stop treatment?

The Bach remedies you initially purchase will last for many years, so the initial cost is often the only cost you will incur. It's not an expensive, painful or unpleasant treatment so go ahead and use it as long as you find that it is helping. Go ahead and stop it when you feel that you don't need it anymore because your tics are so mild they aren't bothering you or because your tics have gone into full remission. Of course you can also stop treatment when you feel like you aren't getting results or progress seems to have halted. If you like, you can consult a Bach Flower Practitioner for further assistance before giving up completely. You will not experience any side-effects from discontinuing the treatment. Starting and stopping repeatedly is the normal process of BFTT healing as described above.

Should I expect my tics to disappear completely or only partially?

Anything can happen. As you already know, they may not disappear at all. And yes, they may completely disappear. In some cases, they just become significantly more mild. But here's one very important thing to note: if the tics go away and then return, it's not that BFTT didn't work. It means that you are IN THE MIDDLE of the treatment! Improvement followed by a return of symptoms is the normal course of healing in BFTT.

My doctor said that my tics will wax and wane throughout life or just disappear completely. Why should I use BFTT if doing nothing will work just as well?

If doing nothing is working well for you, then keep doing it. It is the cheapest and easiest "treatment" available for tics. BFTT is for people who find that "doing nothing" is not working for them.

I've tic'd all my life and I'm used to it. So is everyone around me. What would be the point of starting a treatment now?

A 45 year old may be "used to" his life-long bad posture, and it may not really bother him or anyone in his life, but when a simple posture-correcting intervention is invented (like those cool new bluetooth posture-correctors), he may purchase it because he's still interested in looking his best and feeling his best. Similarly, there are people who are always interested in getting as healthy, attractive and happy as they can possibly be even though they're not in a particularly bad place. When such people have mild or moderate chronic tics that don't warrant behavioral or medical intervention, and they learn about BFTT, they may want to give the treatment a shot. This group of people has traditionally "just lived" with their tics because there has not been a simple, safe and effective intervention for them. Now that there is, many will want to see if it can help them "look and feel their best." Why not?

My child's tics are hardly noticeable. BFTT is easy, but it's still a "treatment." I'm concerned that giving remedies to my child will draw his attention to his tics and make him self-conscious about something he isn't worrying about right now. Is it important to treat him anyway?

The presence of tics indicates an imbalance in the system, something akin to a skin rash. Something is off somewhere. Although you certainly don't have to treat his tics if they're not causing him difficulties, keep in mind that tics are only the tip of the iceberg. You may want to treat them. Moreover, people of all ages usually have symptoms of some kind that ARE annoying to them. BFTT is treating those symptoms as well and one of these other symptoms may be the better "selling" point for your treatment protocol. For instance, a child who has nightmares may be more enthused about treating the nightmares than he is about treating a small twitch. He can be offered BFTT to treat his nightmares without mentioning the twitch at all! This way he is saved from focusing on something that he didn't perceive as a problem.

How do I give my child his daytime doses when he is at school?

Sometimes the remedy needs to be taken when a person is away from home (at school, work, traveling, etc.). In this case, a regular 16-ounce water bottle may be filled with 8 drops (twice the regular amount because you have twice the amount of liquid) and sipped for two separate doses. A child at school might have his first dose of remedy with his breakfast at home and then drink the rest from his prepared water bottle at school during morning recess, some more at lunch time, and the remainder during afternoon recess. He can then have another dose in the early evening. As there is no concept of "overdose" in Bach Treatment, giving your child that fifth dose when he's home from school ensures that treatment continues over the course of a day.

I forgot to take my mid-day dose. It's already 4 pm. Should I just continue with my next two doses as usual?

Sometimes people forget to take their remedy - especially when first starting treatment. In this case, the remedy should be taken whenever the lapse is realized. So if the first dose was taken at 8 am and then at 3 pm the person realizes that the noon dose had been forgotten, a dose can be taken at 3. Then, take two more doses during that day. For example, the next dose could be at 5 pm or 6 pm and the final dose at 8 pm or 9 pm. The important thing is to take four doses a day, separated by some hours. If you realize at 7 pm that you forgot to take the midday dose and your bedtime is 10:30 pm, then there isn't time to take all three remaining doses. In that case, don't worry. Take two doses and tomorrow try again to take four.

I accidentally took an extra dose today. Should I take one less tomorrow?

If you take an extra dose one day, no problem. However, there is no need to take less the following day.

I'm not sure if I've selected the exact remedies that I need. What if I left out something or added something unnecessary. Will BFTT still work?

Some people are concerned that the treatment won't work if they don't choose exactly the right remedies. There is no need for concern. Each remedy is broad-acting. Moreover, if you take a remedy that you don't actually need, it won't cause any harm - it simply won't do anything at all.

My system is very sensitive and I tend to react to any vitamin, herb, food or treatment that I try. When I took my Bach Flower Remedy for the first time tonight, I felt light-headed. Now I'm afraid to take it again.

Remember that the remedies are considered to be medically inactive and are not expected to interact with either allopathic (drugs) or alternative medicines nor produce any side-effects. However, if you've encountered any uncomfortable sensation, including an unusual increase in tics, it is possible that the remedy released a lot of stress in the system very suddenly. The symptom arises because things happened a bit too quickly to be comfortable. In these cases, treatment can be slowed down for the first little while, allowing the body to adjust to stress release more slowly and comfortably. Slowness can be achieved in different ways, depending on the severity of the symptom. If it was a mild reaction, you might take 4 drops just once a day for a few days. If no symptom occurs, then raise that to 4 drops twice a day for another few days. If that goes well, then move it to 4 drops 3 and then 4 times a day in the same way.

If the symptom was intense, then you might just give your body a chance to "meet" the Bach remedies very, very slowly. In this case, I suggest that you reduce the initial treatment to 1 drop once a day, building up to 1 drop twice a day, then 1 drop three times a day, and finally 1 drop four times a day, going as quickly or as slowly as is comfortable. Then, if all is well, begin the same procedure using two drops; if all continues to go well, repeat with 3 drops and finally 4 drops. The steps can be speeded up or slowed down, depending on your personal comfort level. If you still have concerns, consult with and follow the recommendations of a Bach Flower Practitioner or health care provider.

When I started taking the remedies, my tics got worse. Could the remedies have worsened my condition?

Occasionally, symptoms may worsen or new symptoms may appear when a person starts taking Bach remedies. This is known as a "healing reaction." It isn't common with Bach Flower Therapy in general or with BFTT in particular, but it can happen. When it does, follow the suggested protocol for side-effects, described above.

Are Bach Flower Remedies kosher? Can they be used in kosher containers?

Bach Flower Remedies are medicine, not food. They do not require kosher certification. Nonetheless, for kosher consumers who have expressed concern about the presence of grape alcohol as a preservative, Rabbi Pesach Eliyahu Falk, of blessed memory (from Gateshead England), wrote extensively on the permissibility of Bach Flower Remedies as a treatment modality. His ruling states that there is no concern regarding the use of Bach Flower Remedies in kosher vessels or liquids and that they are permissible to take as a regular treatment on the Sabbath and holidays, including Passover.

How long does a Bach remedy last after you purchase it? Can I use a treatment bottle that I prepared a year ago?

There is an expiry date on each bottle, so you can definitely go with that. Alternatively, contact the manufacturer of your product to get your questions answered (Nelson's is the manufacturer of Bach Original Flower Remedies and can be reached at 1-800-319-9151).

Do I Have to Use the Same Mixture All the Time?

No. As you are using the remedies, your symptoms may change. When you mix a new treatment bottle, do it based on the symptoms you are seeing at that time but always include Agrimony. Some people find that the same mixture works again and again, while others find they have one or two "steady" repeat remedies and then a few new ones each time. As long as the remedy fits the way you feel, you should use it. If you are mixing a remedy for a child, the same rule applies. Give the child the remedies for the traits you are seeing now but always add Agrimony.

I'm using BFTT for my child but having learned about the remedies, I'm very interested in using them to treat my anxiety. Can I just make up a treatment bottle for myself using the information you've provided?

Anyone can use Bach Flower Remedies to address their issues. It's as easy as walking into a health food store, reading a description on a pamphlet and taking home some remedies. When there is an emergency requiring urgent medical attention, or emotional symptoms are disrupting functioning at work or at school or are causing great distress, one should see a professional psychological or medical practitioner for assessment and treatment. Otherwise, using self-help techniques is a popular way to help oneself through the stresses of life. If self-help works sufficiently, then that may be all that's needed. There are many forms of self-help besides Bach Flower Remedies. For instance, many people find that learning a breathing technique, taking a yoga class or reading a self-help book is all the help they need to resolve their anxious feelings or low mood. However, there are others who will need much more help in order to address deeper feelings of anxiety or depression. Bach Flower Remedies can be used alone for mild symptoms and stress, or along with professional psychotherapy or medical treatment for more severe symptoms. Similarly, one can continue with one's meditation practice while simultaneously receiving more intensive psychological and/or medical treatment. Bach Flower Remedies can provide emotional support for every member of the family and have been doing so for almost a century!

Where can I learn more about Bach Flower Therapy?

If you'd like more information on the Bach system of healing, you can peruse sites such as bachremedies.com, bachcentre.com, and bach.com, or read one of the many available books on Bach Flower Remedies (my personal favorite is "The Encyclopedia of Bach Flower Therapy" by Mechthild Scheffer).

FINAL THOUGHTS

If you have decided to try BFTT, or if you are still on the fence about proceeding, I want to offer this encouragement: Many people have already been thrilled with the results of their BFTT experiment. Numerous sufferers and parents of sufferers have been enormously grateful for the opportunity to learn about and use this therapeutic modality for their tics. They have found relief without hardship or strain and they've experienced success that they hadn't yet experienced from other treatments. Hopefully, you'll be equally pleased with the results you obtain! I'd love to hear how it goes for you and welcome your feedback. Please share your story with me by sending an email to books@sarahchanaradcliffe.com with the subject line 'No More Tics.'

Wishing you a full and speedy recovery!

Sarah Chana

ABOUT SARAH CHANA RADCLIFFE

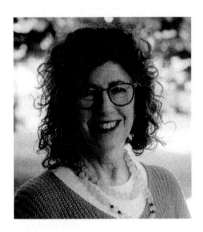

Sarah Chana Radcliffe is a psychologist in Toronto, Canada. She has been helping parents, couples and individuals for more than 40 years. She is the author of "Raise Your Kids without Raising Your Voice," "Better Behavior Now!," "The Fear Fix," "Make Yourself at Home" and numerous other books on family life and emotional stress. She also conducts family-life and stress-management keynotes, workshops and webinars, writes for various online and in-print periodicals, and is a frequent guest on podcasts, blogs and social media sites. Sarah Chana provides education for parents on her Instagram page (instagram.com/sarahchanaradcliffe) and Facebook (facebook.com/scradcliffe), as well as her Daily Parenting Posts email list (dailyparentingposts.com).

Printed in Great Britain
by Amazon

87129163R00038